Eating for Meaning Guide to Detox

Dr. Millie Lytle, ND, CNS

Guide to Detox

DEDICATION

To Tom McCauley and Justine Lynch for building Mountain. Thank you for welcoming me and allowing me to create my program in your sacred space.

CONTENTS

Guide to Detox

ACKNOWLEDGMENTS

Thanks to the motivators in my life. My family, friends, colleagues, and everyone who has put knowledge of body and spirit together to promote peace and wellbeing.

Guide to Detox

1 EATING FOR MEANING

We live in a toxic world. And while our body is constantly detoxing, the chemical burden upon us from our environment is too great to ignore. Regulated and unregulated chemicals are in our food, water, air, soil, medications, canned foods, sugar, alcohol, cleaning products and personal cosmetics. These chemicals make us fat, prematurely old, allergic, autoimmune and may even give us cancer. This is the age of the cancer epidemic but also it's the age of information technology and the age of knowledge. Knowing we can proactively reduce our cancer risk by using age-old tips of detox to improve the efficiency and effectiveness of waste removal from our system is a win-win. It makes you healthier and more beautiful. We detox daily, but let's help our bodies do what they know how to do – let's start with an intensive 2 week program.

Eating for Meaning Guide to Detox provides a step-by-step guide to a 14-day modified brown-rice diet. While your body detoxifies daily, if you have hidden sources of inflammation, suffer from constipation, pain, arthritis, obesity or just feel blah, then a detox is a great way to kick start your metabolism. This terrific cleanse incorporates an optional 1-3 days of liquid fast, plus recipes for salads, dips, breakfast and drinks that are recommended on a cleanse. Cleansing for the first time can be an intense little adventure that will crash course you into understanding how your body uses food. Change up your diet for 2 weeks! See how you feel. See how much weight you lose. How much energy you have. How your symptoms disappear. See how much you learn about yourself! See how pretty you look and how good you feel! How your skin glows!

Eating for Meaning asks you to pay attention to the relationship you have with food such as

- what foods you crave

- what drives you to eat and not to eat

- when to eat and when not to eat

- how you break and continue the cycle of illness

- paying attention to the voice inside to guide you on your food choices

Eating for Meaning relies on 4 principles to guide you to towards making the best choices in the foods you eat. Eating for Meaning uses guidelines because some foods are right for you and wrong for others in your life. The same foods are not healthy for everyone. For example, an apple is a healthy food, but if it causes heartburn, mouth tingling and diarrhea, it is not a healthy food for you. Every time you eat you have an opportunity to choose foods that are making you healthy and energized or foods that are making you overweight and sluggish. The most important principles to guide your towards making the best decisions are yours to make. They are as important as remembering your N.A.M.E.

1) N=Nutrition. This means a variety of things to different people. In this case, I am referring to whole foods nutrition. Eating foods that come from a farm or a garden. They have not been packaged or processed in a plant. They require you to cook them at home. If you order them in a restaurant, you can recognize them from a farm.

You are embarking on the adventure of detox. This might be completely different from the foods you normally eat. It's a very simple diet, easy on the digestion and minimal allergens. There is no refined sugar or salt, no alcohol, no white vinegar, no pepper sauce therefore no condiments. You spice your food through garlic, onions, fresh herbs and fresh ingredients. The adventure is in the preparation. It's a very plain diet and a very repetitive diet. By trying the recipes in chapter 7, you will be on your way towards adventure. I think you will love the way it makes you feel!

The best foods to eat on a detox are foods that improve detoxification and elimination. We call these liver foods. They are beets, green vegetables, lemons, garlic, onions, organic green apples, grapefruit, broccoli family vegetables such as cauliflower, cabbage, bok choy, watercress, arugula, mustard greens, kohlrabi, broccoli rabe, rapini, kale, collard greens, turnip, and of course broccoli. We can increase the intensity and effectiveness of a detox by including appropriate supplements, located on page 47.

Using this guide we will re-create the gene-resetting detox diet. There is an optional fast within with cleanse. See the chapter on Detox waters for the fasting portion of the cleanse. You can stretch this out or keep it short to 3 days. The most effective fast is to consume 0 to 400 calories per day. I have also included the option of a mono diet.

2) A=Adventure. The joy of eating is almost as important as the food itself. It's important to enjoy, explore, experiment and cook. It's only by preparing food ourselves, with our loved ones and for others that we truly become connected to the adventure of food. Finding new foods outside our comfort zone is another key to introducing variety into our diets.

The adventure of a detox is trying out something new for yourself. Eating for health and wellness alone. Eating to make change. Eating to find a new way. Eating to learn more about you. You may try foods you've never had before. This diet may send you to some new stores, some new restaurants or keep you home instead of going out. You will surely benefit from making a brief but life-lasting change. It IS truly Adventurous to do a cleanse.

3) M=Mindfulness is about paying attention to the way food makes you feel. Not only focusing on how tasty the food is, but also the texture, the energy, the cleanliness, and the energy of the food, particularly if it gives you energy or robs you of energy. Food has calories. Calories are energy, so they should not make you want to sleep after eating them. Likewise, food should not make you sick to your stomach, heartburn, itchy, indigestion or depressed.

The period of detox is all about paying attention to how you feel now that all the nasty and toxic food is out of your diet. You might notice you have less energy for a couple days then a lot of energy. You may feel withdrawal or hangover symptoms. You may have good bowel movements. You may have a skin outbreak, after 3 days, your skin gets glowing. Your moods become stable. You don't have sugar highs and lows. You are paying attention to everything you eat to the minute details as well as focusing on how you feel about the food you eat and what you observe in your body. This is YOU time!

4)   E=Epigenetics is the science of understanding that the behavior of genes depends on their environment. You are born with a set of genes inherited by your mother, father and ancestors. While the presence of these genes may be fixed, the behavior of these genes is not. In fact, genes can remain off towards youth or on towards chronic disease.

By fasting for 3 days without any calories, AND by eating 1200 calories per day of low calorie, high nutrient superfoods only (salad leaves, berries, seeds, seaweeds and cruciferous family vegetables) you can reset your genes. You will reduce genetic related conditions from expressing themselves, you will prevent passing down inherited genes to your children, you will lower your cancer risk.

Some foods you may have thought are healthy are common allergens. They might be making you sick. A modified brown rice diet is beneficial as it combines low allergy whole foods with a clean diet, mostly prepared by you. It incorporates the temporary removal of highly allergenic foods such as wheat gluten, orange juice, soy, peanuts, dairy, vinegar and packaged/canned foods. It prioritizes the removal of alcohol, sugar and processed foods. Once the detox is over, I recommend strategically reintroducing foods so you can continue to learn about the foods that are not right for you.

Let's break this down by looking at 8 detox benefits that may make you begin right away.

•   You will lose weight very easily at first. Your body stores up a lot of waste that can only be released through a good detox program, like THIS ONE! Perhaps you have tried different diets and have lost weight temporarily. The reason for that is because the toxins are still in your system which can easily trigger cravings that you have for unhealthy food.

Before you make any kind of dietary lifestyle changes, you can detox so you will not go back to unhealthy eating habits.

- You will reduce the amount of toxins and pollutant within your body, thus lessening the burden against the detoxification organs. Your organs will work much better, they will be healthier and as a result, you will feel be much healthier as well.

- It will strengthen your bodies fight against cancer cells and also allow generation of healthy cells. Cancer cells are bred by toxins and once it is all eliminated, the odds of you never facing cancer will be that much greater.

- Your immune system will be greatly improved. You will find that after detoxing, you may not catch the latest bug or cold that is going around. Or even if you do, you will fight it off very quick because your immune system will be so much stronger.

- You will feel more mentally alert and not so tired all the time. Your brain will be working more effectively and efficiently because of those toxins being gone.

- Although you may get a breakout at the start of a detox, after a few days your skin will look better and be much more healthy. You will not be prone to blemishes or other skin conditions after detoxing as well.

- A good detox benefits your life expectancy, with the reduced stress on the detoxification organs such as the liver, bowel and kidneys.

- You will find you'll have a lot more energy. The sluggishness you constantly feel is due to toxins weighing you down. You know how you feel exhausted after eating a high carb meal? That's your body telling you that food robs you of energy. When detoxing those moments will disappear.

Your body and mind will be much healthier than before. With a toxin free body, the work rate will be significantly reduced by it having to try and fight against all the pollutants that were in it before. The body can then concentrate on more important tasks such as restoring your body and fighting against degenerative and chronic diseases.

These are just some of the detox benefits that you will see after going through a detox program. When done properly they can rejuvenate your body and mind and make you feel like a new person. Detox benefits are very apparent and results easy to achieve, it just takes some expert guidance to determine the best detox for you.

Change up your diet for 2 weeks! See how you feel. See how much weight you lose. See how much you learn about yourself! You will feel better and lose weight on this diet.

2 CONCEPTS OF DETOX

The main concept of a detox is to give your body a break by consuming simple foods without as few toxins as possible. To eat clean for two weeks allows your digestion a chance to catch up and heal from various food decisions, parties, bouts of indigestion, flares up and other chronic symptoms that bad food choices can ignite. A detox also provides an opportunity to reset you metabolism and kick off a weight loss program. When you go on a detox, you are eating low calorie foods that have been prepared in a simple way without the use of condiments, sugar, spices and salts. You are also weeding out food allergens and sensitivities. So if you need to determine which foods are making you sick this diet allows you to do that quickly and efficiently by removing the most common food allergens. By doing this you will generally feel better but become more responsive to the foods that are bad for you. Buyer beware, once you go on a detox, you WILL learn if milk, cheese, beer, pasta, bread and wine are bad for you, once and for all! Likely you will be forever changed. Lastly, you are also resetting your genes, reducing hormones levels that might cause diabetes, high blood pressure, autoimmune conditions, obesity and even cancers.

Studies show that your genetic predisposition towards chronic disease can be reset by eating a calorie restricted diet. This means you can lower your risk of common illness such as cancer, Alzheimer's, Diabetes can be reset by fasting. Studies show that a 1200 calories per day diet, rich in plant foods like seeds, greens, berries and other naturally low-calories wonder-foods can lower your risk for illness, keep you lean and younger than the rest of your friends. You can achieve the same effect by fasting; consuming 0 calories and only water and herbal teas for 3 days. This is how you reset your genes towards health and away from chronic illness; with nutrition.

NOTE: If you already have a chronic illness such as heart disease or diabetes you may not be able to follow the fast, in which case you continue the brown rice diet detox. Systematically lowering caloric intake to 1200 kcals/day will also reset your genes in the long run. Studies show that therapeutic calorie restrictors who eat all the required nutrients in fewer calories age more slowly and develop less chronic disease.

To succeed at this cleanse. Do groceries prior to the start so you have plenty to eat. This diet is under the guidance of myself, Dr. Millie. If you'd like one-on-one consultation, be in touch before you start the detox. I will need to know all your health concerns prior to starting.

Foods with highest nutrients in the fewest calories- Under 40 calories per serving (1/2 cup) and jam packed with nutrition: This means you could eat your weight in these foods per day and never gain a pound! In fact, have you ever heard about the foods that take more calories to eat than they contain? THESE ARE THEM!!!!!!! These foods actually cause you to burn more calories than they provide. Plus they are filled with energizing nutrients for your brain, nervous system. Plus, they are all friendly to diabetes, cancer,

1 cup of brown rice has 215 calories and 1 cup of cooked quinoa has 223 calories. 1 cup of any of the foods below have 50 or fewer calories. If you eat 2.5-3 cups of brown rice or quinoa per day, 2 servings of any of these foods at each meal and another 100 calorie snack, you will be within a therapeutic calorie restriction diet (<1200 calories). Plus, it's a lot of food.

22 Best Detox Foods:

- Arugula

- Asparagus

- Beets

- Berries (except strawberry)

- Bone Broth

- Broccoli

- Brussels sprouts

- Cabbage

- Carrots

- Cauliflower

- Celery

- Cocoa (raw or pure, free of sugar and milk)

- Fennel

- Grapefruit

- Kale

- Lettuce

- Peppers

- Pumpkin

- Radish

- Tomato

- Watercress

- Zucchini

Garlic, onions, lemons, limes, coffee, cocoa, Broth, herbal tea, fresh green or organic carrot juice, tea green round out the foods on the detox.

The majority of nutritionists and dieticians who you consult on changing your diet will focus on weight loss. After all, who doesn't want to look their best, right? These knowledgeable health lovers will give you detailed exercises to do, and provide you a list of foods that are considered healthy. They may even recommend herbs, juicing, blending and supplements. They will give you lots of pep talks as well. Out of consideration for your own comfort, they will always tell you that it's all right to go easy on yourself once in a while and give in to that delicious treat.

However, here is the reality. When detoxing, your body is especially sensitive to bad food. This same bad food that is considered toxic will also cause obesity but while on a cleanse will cause more immediate reactions as well. If you have a very unhealthy lifestyle that consists of foods that are toxic, your overall health will be in danger. You will be prone to illnesses such as cancer, diabetes, and your immune system will be quite low if your diet consists of processed food and other junk. If you eat these foods while detoxing you will be more likely to suffer negative effects such as skin rash, nausea, IBS, stress, lack of sleep and an overall toxic feeling. No matter which detox you choose this fall be sure you are not consuming poisons at the same time.

Below are listed the top 10 toxic foods to avoid on a detox.

1. **Alcohol**– Not only does alcohol contain twice as many calories as fatty foods, too much also leads to a host of other health and psychological. Alcohol is the main culprit for conditions like cirrhosis. While small amounts of alcohol from a healthy source, like organic red grapes may help with circulatory health, alcohol itself is a toxic to the liver. It also depletes the body of essential nutrients. It also promote estrogen-like behaviors and can increase risk of breast, prostate and ovarian cancers.

2. **Caffeine**– so caffeine is not really a food! Coffee, tea and energy drinks all contain this liver and neurotoxin. Depending on the source a small amount of caffeine is not bad. In unsweetened organic green tea and fair trade espresso a cup while on a detox is sometimes allowed. Better to focus on naturally decaffeinated lemon water, herbal teas and pure spring water.

3. **White Bread** is a processed food from another processed food, bleached white flour. In addition to lacking nutrients, fiber and having the same glycemic index as sugar, white bread also has other forbidden ingredients such as yeast. A definite hazard while on a detox. And whole wheat bread is not much better and in some cases worse, due to added sugars! This includes bagels, pastries, pasta, wheat bread with enriched white flour in it, cakes, cookies, crackers and saltines.

4. **Sugar**– Especially when it is processed like high fructose corn syrup. However all toxic bleached white sugar whether from corn, sugar beet or sugarcane are filled with bleach, pesticides. They are habit forming, mood and immune weakening! It is a simple sugar that makes you gain weight fast as well, interrupts hormone cycles, promotes diabetes, cancer and cravings. It also promotes the growth of bacteria, yeast and reduces the ability of your immune system to fight.

5. **Dairy Products**– These products that come from cows given growth hormones and antibiotics are certainly toxic. You are getting disgusting medicine with every gulp. Even organic dairy products, which unfortunately

includes cheese and ice cream but also otherwise healthy foods such a cottage cheese, butter and milk are a no-no while on a detox. Reason being, they cause mucous, fatigue and yeast overgrowth. Yes, even most yogurts on the market are more likely to generate bad critters than prevent them. The fat content doesn't make a difference. The good news is nut, grain and bean milks, as long as they are organic and unsweetened are allowed.

6. **Fast Food**– Major fast food chains use pre-made, factory farmed meat that is highly processed. They use white bread that is also very processed. Everything that you will find at a fast food restaurant is overcooked, deep fried, overly salted and cooked in rancid oils. The next time you are hungry and have a craving to get a meal from any major fast food chain, you will want to think twice on that, even when NOT on a detox.

7. **Junk Food**– Another word for that is "wanna be food". Think of candy, microwavable foods, fruit drinks (not juice) such as Kool-Aid, Tang and then there are confections such as marshmallows, chips, cheezies, and all sugared children's cereals definitely all fall into this category. This is your opportunity to kick that toxic microwaveable popcorn once and for all! Chips are in fact healthier than microwaveable popcorn. If you must eat popcorn, switch to organic, stove top pop or air pop. Just make sure your popping corn is organic because GMO is a NO-GO.

8. **GMO**– Genetically modified crops include soy, corn (some sweet corn), sugar(beet), canola, cotton, some zucchinis, squashes and Hawaiian papaya. All foods made with these ingredients , unless organic or specifically say "non-gmo" are resistant to pesticides because they produce a virus that is "Round Up Ready" or "Round Up Resistant". Yes, the plant itself is making a toxic chemical that cannot be washed off and it requires more pesticide sprayed on it. The World Health Organization has admitted that the pesticide Round Up is likely carcinogenic. Many other countries have banned the import of American GMOs crops concerned for their endocrine disrupting hazards. Endocrine disruptors can affect puberty, appetite, fertility and increase cancer risk.

9. **Canned Food**– While in a pinch canned tuna, salmon or lentils might be an okay option, foods preserved in canned are pressure heated leaving behind very few nutrients. Think canned peas! Are they even edible? The second problem is the lining of the can itself seeps into the food. This lining contain cancer-causing estrogen mimickers called pthalates and Bisphenol A. It's surely a good idea to avoid these and prepare you beans and veggies from scratch.

10. **BBQ Meat**– No meat is truly detoxifying and not recommended on a detox. However meat cooked at high temperatures on the grill, BBQ or fryer are worse. This meat flesh becomes slowly burned, charred or caramelized leaving behind cancer and Alzheimers-causing proteins called polycyclic aromatic hydrocarbons and heterocyclic amines.

3 ORGAN DETOX

The body's six emunctories are: the liver, kidney, lungs, skin, colon and gall bladder. I will briefly go over each organ's cleansing role.

- **The Liver–** This powerful organ cleans the blood and conjugates harmful chemicals for excretion. It Lords over all toxins of the body by cleaning all the body's blood and metabolizing all chemicals, even the good kind. First the liver takes toxins and converts them to smaller molecules then it renders them safe for excretion by neutralizing them and package them up for elimination. The liver also makes bile, cholesterol and stores vitamins like D, A and B12. When the liver is stressed it shows elevated liver enzymes. But a fatty liver, right side tenderness, high cholesterol, indigestion and constipation can all be signs the liver is not up to par, and needs some help. Detox the liver with bitter herbs, foods and facilitating the body's production of glutathione with supplements.

- **The Kidneys–** The role of the kidney is that it flushes waste and toxins from your blood, once it's cleaned by the liver. The kidneys flush water soluble waste in response to water and electrolyte concentrations. At least 2 quarts of water is recommended daily on a cleanse. Greens herbs and teas are weak diuretics that promote kidney detox. Parsley, cilantro, green tea, nettle and alfalfa are great for flushing the kidney and reduce blood pressure in the kidney. Cranberry and juniper berry are good renal tonics to flush extra toxins and prevent bacteria build up in the kidney.

- **The Lungs–** Your lungs are responsible for filtering out CO_2, fumes, mold, allergens, and airborne toxins. Just by breathing expiring deeply you are detoxing your lungs. Sleeping soundly without sleep apnea or excessive snoring also promotes lung detox. Use a Himalayan salt pipe or go to the beach to breathe in salt air in order to clean the lungs further. Remember the more pollution you inhale through smoking the more you are making your lungs toxic. Many herbs and nutrients can also detoxify the lungs N-Acetyl-Cysteine, Black Seed, Rosemary, Lobelia, Pleurisy Root and Chrysanthemum are all excellent for lung health.

- **The Lymph**- The lymphatic system parallels your red blood circulation and removes products of infection, bacteria, virus and other pathogens from the circulation. Lymph nodes can become tender and swollen as a result of infection being cleared. Non tender lymph are a sign of stagnation, that the lymph system is not clearing waste. It can be a sign of cancer. The lymph system requires movement in order to function well. You can promote lymph movement by tapping on your thymus gland 10 times. The thymus gland sits under the breast bone, at the nipple line in the center of your chest. You can also promote lymph detoxify by gently using a natural bristle brush or sea sponge and brushing your skin in circular motion from your feet up to your heart, from your neck and finger tips up to your heart. Do it before showering for extra benefit. Exercise and breast massage also promote lymph detox. Movement is key.

- **Skin**– Its role is to sweat out toxins. Like your lungs, it can absorb waste and then release it through salty sweat and release of heat. To be honest we don't know all the waste products that are absorbed into the skin or released from the skin. But we do know the skin is our largest organ, always exchanging oxygen and waste. All forms of detox benefit the skin particularly exercise, dry skin brushing and saunas. The skin wants to sweat at key times of day. Remember to rehydrate.

- **Colon**– Its job is to excrete chemical waste, so it is not re-circulated into the bloodstream. It also houses protective bacteria called microbiome. In order for the colon to detox it needs to get rid of pounds of old stool, which half of Americans have in abundance. Detox the colon by increasing soluble and insoluble fibers, edible bentonite clay, probiotics and herbal or salt laxatives. If you are fasting and not consuming any solid food, the you particularly need to focus on the salt flush in order to eliminate during fasting days.

- **Gallbladder—** This organ releases bile, a detergent for your body's fat and cholesterol metabolism. Bile washes the fat away. The gall bladder responds to fats, so it's important to have olive oil and coconut oil on the diet. You can give your gall bladder a flush by eating 6-8 organic apples in one day; do the mono diet to soften small stones or sludge and then do the **Gallbladder Flush: Before bed, mix 1/2 cup olive oil and 1/2 cup fresh squeezed lemon juice and drinking it before bed. Lay on your right side.**

Even though these emunctories naturally cleanse, with all of the pollution and toxins around, and our bad diets- they can easily become overloaded and fail to work properly.

For instance, if your bowels are not moving on a regular basis (as you should have a bowel movement after each meal), waste will sit in your body. When that happens your health will be impeded and will create toxicity. Especially when it comes to estrogen-by products since estrogen is metabolized in the liver, then excreted by bile into the digestive system. The large bowel or colon has bacteria that breaks down the estrogen even further. If too much estrogen is in your body due to these organs not functioning properly, that will automatically increase your risk for cancer. This is one of many reasons it is crucial to detox your body by doing a cleanse.

A detox program is there to help the functioning of all the detox organs through: fresh food and herbs, pure water, exercise, deep breathing, saunas/sweating and waste excretion so that the body works more efficiently at generating and using energy. Sometimes we think of a detox as spring cleaning! But there are lots of environmental changes going on in the fall too and we are rebalancing our immune systems for the winter months.

Symptoms of Detox:

What is it detoxification? Explanation from NSA Detoxification is the term used to describe the process your body goes through to get rid of toxins. Detoxification symptoms-both physical and mental - may appear when you alter your lifestyle by starting something new, such as changing your diet or exercising, or by discontinuing a current habit, such as eating chocolate or drinking coffee. These symptoms include headache, stomachache, cough, diarrhea, skin eruptions (rash), clogged sinus, and fever, as well as feeling run down and irritable. The symptoms may be of short duration and slight irritation, or they could last longer and cause you considerable discomfort.

Because these symptoms are the same as those that show up in certain illnesses, changing your diet or lifestyle can result in misunderstanding: If I am doing something that is supposed to be good for me, why do I have these symptoms? Why do I feel worse, and not better? Understanding this apparent contradiction is perhaps the first, and most important, hurdle you must get over when making a dietary or lifestyle change. If you consider this contradiction carefully, however, it is easy to understand. Think of how you might have experienced this on a short-term basis. If you do not get regular exercise and then play some softball with your kids, the next day you might feel bad - tired with sore muscles. This is your body reacting to something that it is not used to doing. You can see the same thing when you stop a regular activity; if you are a soda drinker and stop drinking soda for a while, you may notice that you have less energy and you may even have a headache. When you change your diet or lifestyle, the same thing happens; your body reacts to the change.

Why does this happen? As we live, toxins accumulate in our bodies. Some of these are due to our diet and others are due to the environment around us. Of course, our lifestyle also fits in - if you smoke or use alcohol you are accumulating even more toxins. When you make a change in diet or lifestyle, through stopping a bad habit or eating better, your cells begin to eliminate the toxic substances. Before finding the exit, however, the toxins are released into the bloodstream and are carried through the circulatory system. This transportation and elimination may result in headache, diarrhea, or constipation, and often toxins are eliminated through the skin, resulting in rashes or skin problems (especially if you are prone to such problems). You may also feel a lack of energy, especially if you are eliminating meats from your diet. (The protein found in meat is more stimulating than that found in vegetables.)

You may also find that, with the absence of toxins, you absorb substances more easily. Thus, the sugar and caffeine in a soda might really set you off. In a nutshell, we could say that the body always goes for quality, and when the food coming in is of higher quality than the present tissue, the body will discard the present tissue because it wants to make room for tissue created by the higher-quality food. How severe are the symptoms and how long do they last? How long the symptoms last and how severe they are depend on your lifestyle before making a change and how quickly you make a change. If you have a diet heavy in red meats, for example, and become a vegetarian overnight, you might have severe symptoms for a time. If your lifestyle changes are gradual, the symptoms could be less severe. The duration of the symptoms might not be linear; there is a greater chance that they will come in cycles. At first you may feel great and then experience some detoxification symptoms. After the initial toxins are flooded out, you will feel good again, if not better. However, the body "goes deeper" and finds more toxins to eliminate; the symptoms may reappear again, and after more toxins are eliminated, you will feel better yet. As things progress, you will find that the period of symptoms is shorter and the period of well-being greater. What can I do during this period?

The hardest thing for many people to do is accept that they are not sick and realize that the body is cleansing itself. Once you get beyond this psychological barrier, the rest is easy. The most important thing to do can be summed up in one word: Rest. Rest, and let the body do what it needs to. If you have the luxury of staying home, do so! If not, cut back on social engagements and perhaps even cut back on any exercise you are getting. Give your body as much energy as possible to do its jobs. Eat light foods that are easy to digest - consume fruits and vegetables and drink plenty of water.
Some Possible Detoxification Symptoms:

Guide to Detox

Clogged Skin	Fever	Moodiness
Constipation	Cold Symptoms	Skin breakouts
Cough	Gas	Rash
Diarrhea	Headache	Stomach ache
Fatigue	Irritability	

4 MODIFIED BROWN RICE DIET

EFM 14 DAY DETOX WITH 3 DAY FAST (OR MONO DIET)

General Instructions:
This diet will give you all the nutrition that you will need while your body cleanses and heals itself. You don't have to go hungry, and you don't' have to count calories, weigh food, or pay attention to the selection of food. You eat whenever you are hungry, and as often as you like. While on this diet, you may experience some weight loss.

Eat until you feel full, but not engorged. It is better to eat several small meals per day rather than 3 large ones.

Do not drink with your meals, as this dilutes the enzymes in the stomach needed to properly digest the food eaten. Wait about 10 to 15 minutes before or after eating to drink.
Try to keep the consumption of fruits separate from vegetables and rice. Food combining is based on the discovery that certain combinations of foods may be digested with greater ease and efficiency than others. Therefore, eat only fruits at one time, vegetables and rice at another time. This goes for fruit and vegetable juices as well. Some will even separate rice and vegetables, but this is extreme.

During a cleanse, many individuals can be uncomfortable and tired. If this is happening to you usually it goes away after 3 days. I recommend to hang in there until the program is complete. After a cleanse, you will always feel more energetic, lighter, and you will even be happier overall due to good food, lots of water, movement and feeling great.

Exceptions: eat the foods below, but if you suspect you have a sensitivity to any of them, OR if you react to any of them while on the detox, eliminate them immediately and add them into the rotation.

FROM DAY 1-14: EAT ONLY THESE FOODS: (and as much as you like!)
* **ORGANIC BROWN RICE** What's allowed on the diet?
1)   Brown rice, short grain, long grain, basmati, preferably

organic, quinoa and millet

Cooking Instructions for Brown rice:
Rinse the rice well, 5 or six times in warm water. Proportions of water to rice for cooking are 2-2 1/2 cups of water to 1 cup of rice. Bring water to a boil, add the rice, stir, cover and reduce heat to simmer for 45 minutes, or until all the water has been absorbed. Do not lift the lid until cooking is finished, after which the rice will be doubled in volume and fluffy looking.

Alternate Method:
Rinse rice as above. Bring pot of water to boil, as when cooking pasta. Add desired amount of rice. Allow to boil with lid off until rice becomes soft. Drain water, cover with lid, and allow to steam 5 minutes.

Onions, herbs or spices can be added if desired during the last 15-20 minutes of cooking time.

VEGETABLES (organic preferably, but these are difficult to find)

All kinds of whole vegetables can be eaten (except for corn and white potatoes). Make sure to wash them very well. They can be eaten raw, steamed or baked. Combine them with rice if you wish. No frozen, canned or jarred vegetables should be eaten. Fresh vegetables, any kind you like, lightly steamed. Onions are especially good for cleansing and are very sweet and tasty when steamed. Try a plate full with some fresh garlic.

FRUITS (organic! Especially when it comes to the dirty dozen)

Many kinds of whole fruits can be eaten : preferably grapefruit, apples, pears, pomegranates, kiwi, blueberries, blackberries, raspberries
(rule out bananas, strawberries, oranges, orange juice, melons and dried fruit [mostly because they are treated with sulfates, a food additive allergen]).
Make sure to wash fruit very well. Eat fruit raw. Eat fruit by itself: 1/2 hour before or 2 hours after a meal. Wash very thoroughly especially if not organic with vinegar. Rinse well.

How to tell if it's organic, conventional or frankenfood:
Code begins with 4 = conventional, sprayed with chemical pesticides
Begins with 9= organic, not sprayed with chemical pesticides though can be sprayed with natural pesticides

Begins with a 3 or 8= test crops, Frankenfoods and genetically engineered. Not necessarily sprayed with more pesticides than conventional but not organic

The Dirty Dozen are the fruits and veggies that are most contaminated with pesticides. The list, comprised by the Environmental Working Group change yearly, but generally they remain the same: Here is the list for 2015: Only choose organics of the following:
apples, peaches, nectarines, strawberries, grapes, celery, spinach, sweet bell peppers, cucumbers, cherry tomatoes, imported snap peas and potatoes. Salad greens, kale and collards are also heavily contaminated.

Likewise **The Clean Fifteen** are the safest conventional fruits and veggies. Here is the 2015 list:
Avocados were the cleanest, non GMO sweet corn, pineapples, cabbage, frozen sweet peas, onions, asparagus, mangoes, papayas, kiwis, eggplant, grapefruit, cantaloupe, cauliflower and sweet potatoes

CONDIMENTS (Very Few!)

Olive/Flax/Coconut oils, fresh lemon/lime juice,* cayenne pepper, herbs and spices that contain no salt or MSG like fresh basil, parsley, turmeric, cinnamon, ginger, cilantro, garlic,
- Himalayan, Real or Celtic sea salt ok
- sauerkraut with salt only, kimchi, apple cider vinegar,
- Other foods allowed are lentils, seaweeds (no MSG) rice cakes, sesame seeds, humus, organic tofu, and tempeh if extra protein is needed.
- Lentils, peas, chickpeas, mung beans, dried, soaked and cooked or sprouted. All varieties. Beans dips and hummus
- Raw or lightly toasted seeds and nuts; flax, chia, pumpkin, walnuts, hemp, almonds, and their butters – 1-2 handfuls at a time.
- Avocado oil

(Avoid cashews, peanuts, macadamia nuts, pecans)

*Flaxseed oil (this oil must be refrigerated, never heated and used within 3 weeks of opening it)

Vegetable and fruit juice –preferably cold pressed organic- the best is fresh pressed from a juicer, otherwise juices with no additives, sugar, chemicals, and little or no salt (can be found in health food stores)

Non Detox Foods: Stay away from foods high on food chain. (if necessary: ocean-going fish, organic eggs)

BEVERAGES (Mostly water!)
Filtered distilled or spring water. *Herbal teas, such as milk thistle, dandelion leaf and root, licorice root, green tea, blueberry leaf, bilberry, rooibos, organic green tea, etc. Pure pomegranate, cranberry and blueberry juices. *Vegetable and fruit juices – preferably freshly made and organic. However, if they are from jars or cans, make sure they contain nothing other than 100% juice. (Read your labels). Dilute juices with water half and half.
Drink liquids ½ hour before or 1 hour after eating
OTHER INSTRUCTIONS:
This is your cleanse, so you can make a mistake or an exception, bug get back on
Follow instructions on supplements.
If you choose to fast or follow a mono diet, stop eating this diet on day 6 and resume on day 11.
Fasting diet starts day 7-10.
*These foods can be found at your local health food store, alternative grocers or health food section of supermarkets
OPTIONAL FASTING: DAY 7-10:
Option 1:
Periodic Fasting: The fastest way to lower chronic disease risk may be periodic fasting. Please note, this is only for those whose current level of health allows for this. Consult your doctor and do this only under Dr. Millie's supervision. Research shows that 3 days of fasting (consuming 0 calories) lowers Insulin Growth Factor, a promoter of chronic illness and premature aging.
Here's how you do it to quickly reset genes:
Starting on Day 7: 3 DAY Fast: Drink only water and Detox waters for 3 days. The best options are 0 calorie herbal teas and salt sole. No sugar or sweetener will keep these waters calorie free. The master cleanse, various juices, broths and grain coffees are also an option
If you are going to select this option, it's necessary to do the salt flush or detox tea/rhubarb/cascara segrada/laxative tea to maintain bowel movements in the absence of solid food.

Option 2:
The Mono Diet intensifies your detox, gives your organs a further break and cleanses your system more deeply. It likely will reset some genes.

Starting on Day 7:
The Mono Diet intensifies your detox, gives your organs a further break and cleanses your system more deeply. It likely will reset some genes.

Starting on Day 7: 3 Day Mono Diet: Eat as much as you like: raw or cooked cabbage and onions and green apples, water and herbal teas (no sugar). Some of you might be getting ready to do some Mono Diets: Choose a vegetable and choose a fruit. Eat the food, raw, steamed, boiled, in broth, juiced or blended.

No other food is to be added, such as salt, oil or seasonings.

Breakfast and Dinner

- Eating nothing but Cabbage, cauliflower, broccoli or asparagus for breakfast and dinner.
- If wanting to add a second vegetable – add steamed or boiled onions

Lunch
- Eating nothing but grapefruit, apples, blackberries, watermelon, for lunch.

Here are some Benefits to Mono Diets, besides the obvious of weight loss:

-resetting your genes to reduce cancer causing insulin growth factor
-Very easy to digest
-It increases detox
-Makes it easier to find out what foods you're sensitive to
-It forces you to eat better quality foods
- It's a very simple way to eat - raw, steamed or in boiled water, but no other ingredients

-It increases appreciation for food, you can savor the food, etc.
- helps you make better decision about being full
- spiritual reasons – it puts you in touch with all other relational aspects of how, when, what you eat. What connections you draw like hunger, boredom, when you're full

Option 3:

Liquid Diet: Drink nothing but fluids for 1-3 days

1) Master Cleanser: Organic Grade C (or Organic B Maple Syrup is next best), Organic Fresh Lemon Juice, Cayenne Pepper, Spring or Filtered Water. Approximately 2 tablespoons of each per quart (32 ounces) of water.

2) Green and veggie juices; not blended, just veggie or mixed veggie and fruit combinations with garlic, ginger, lemon, cucumber, organic celery, organic carrots, organic beets, etc. Juice must be all organic.

Option 4: can be done in conjunction with the mono diet

For the **Gallbladder Flush – if you have gallbladder pain or stones**

- Eat apples alone (about 10 organic green apples or drink only fresh pressed apple juice) for one day.
- Before bed, mix 1/2 cup olive oil and 1/2 cup fresh squeezed lemon juice and drinking it before bed.
- Lay on your right side with your left leg elevated

Day 11 Drink water only (optional)
Day 12 resume the detox diet

NOTES: After the initial 10-14 days, it is important to come off the diet gradually. Don't overeat or splurge on junk food.

Continue through Day 14. This diet can be a very difficult venture if you are not prepared. You must have the food in your cupboards and know where you can eat outside. The more you stick with it, the better you will feel. Try your best and concentrate on what you are able to do, not what you aren't able to.

5 MOST FILLING DETOX FOODS

Some of the best foods that detox the body contain lots of properties that are not only good for helping your body to flush out unwanted toxins, but can also make you feel full. Sounds great doesn't it? It sure is, but you will be surprised to know that the majority of people do not know about this and as a consequence, don't benefit from them. Fortunately, I am about to try and change that for you now and give you some absolute great free tips on how you can easily and safely boost your body's toxin removal system.

Keep in mind of one thing. When you are undergoing any kind of detox program, you are drastically changing your diet and the last thing you are going to want to feel is ravenously hungry. Because if you are starving and edgy, you will have more food cravings and not likely stick with it. If you don't stick with the program, then all of your detoxing efforts from even a few days ago could be gone. Listed below are 10 filling detox foods you will want to munch on while going through the detox program. All of them are under 50 calories so while they are filling, they help weight loss, metabolism. These foods are nutrient dense therefore have a lot of bang for your buck.

Asparagus – Not only does it help to detoxify the body, it can help you wage the anti-aging battle, protect you from getting cancer, help your heart to stay healthy, and is a general anti-inflammatory food. The green leafy spear is wonderful for your kidney and can even help alleviate kidney stones. It's called the Asparagus cure. Plus, asparagus contains only 3 calories per spear or 27 calories per cup

Beets– Beets contain a group of phytonutrients called betalains that support liver detoxification and literally push out toxins. Many people think beets are high in sugar, they do taste earthy and sweet, but in fact 1/2 cup of beets contains only 29 calories. That means a whopping two cups of beets (SO FILLING) is under 120 calories. There ain't no Special K bar that will fill you like 2 cups of beets.

Yukon gold potatoes (boiled and cooled)– This may surprise many since potatoes are known to be starchy. However, this Canadian hybrid potato when boiled and cooled, is excellent for staying full on a detox. A 1/4 cup of boiled YG potato only has 35 calories. The yellow pigment of a Yukon Gold potato is caused by carotenoids, a type of antioxidant. Antioxidants neutralize free radicals and may strengthen the immune system and protect against some forms of cancer. Also cold boiled potatoes have a starch resistant fiber in them which is great for blood sugar stability. Yukon gold potatoes are not nightshades so don't cause inflammation and joint pain, associated with other white and red skin potatoes.

Broccoli – A cruciferous vegetable, broccoli has phytonutrient glucoraphanin which, when converted to *sulforaphane* can boost the livers detoxification enzymes to clear estrogenic and plastic substances that are known to cause cancer. Is it any surprise that 1 cup of cooked broccoli has only 28 calories?

Broth – Commercial based broth is not ideal for detoxing. In fact, they are usually full of salt and MSG which defeats the purpose. However, homemade broth, without any calories, can be full of nutrients, minerals, and electrolytes to keep your blood pressure stable while detoxing. See recipe for Potassium Broth. Quick way: When you steam or simmer any organic veggies, drink the water! Instant broth.

Pumpkin – Pumpkins contain properties which can help for weight loss, increased immune function, and can help heal your skin too due to its rich source of beta carotenoids. Another veggie we equate with richness. Pumpkin pie, right? Thank goodness pumpkin itself, and other squashes too, are naturally so low in calories, only 30 calories per raw cup, and like beets, 59 calories per cup, when cooked.

Brussels Sprouts – They hold as much as 50 times more antioxidants and enzyme stimulating nutrients than many other vegetables. Like other brassica or cruciferous family of veggies (kale, broccoli, cabbage, cauliflower), they detoxify fat soluble toxins that can lead to cancer and fibroids. Eat up, only 30 calories per 1/2 cup, cooked.

Berries (any kind) -Berries have always been hailed for their medicinal effects. They contain antioxidants and many nutrients that move blood, give a pink glow while cleansing and flushing out toxins from the body. Half a cup of blueberries has just 43 calories so eat up because their fiber content blocks blood sugar uptake.

Carrots– Bugs bunny's favorites clean our insides by scrubbing the walls of the colon, removing dangerous toxins and pulling out unused hormones. Another myth is that carrots have high amounts of sugar, maybe in the juice, but the caloric value of raw carrots is relatively low, 25 cals a piece.

Cabbage – cabbage has cleansing properties due to their high content of glucosinolates, sulfur-containing compounds that are converted into active forms isothiocyanates and indoles. Isothiocyanates may prevent cancer by promoting the elimination of potential carcinogens from the body. Cabbage can be eaten raw or cooked. Is a great food choice on a mono diet, where you are only eating 1-3 foods per day because it is so filling, and yet it only contains 17 calories per raw cup!! Wow! And it's so filling.

Lentils – at 14 calories per tablespoon you can enjoy 1/2 cup of lentils, for a little over a 100 calories. Lentils reduce sugar cravings because they provide blood sugar stability with fiber that sweeps your colon clean of bad cholesterol and old waste. They are also a great source of vegetarian protein. Very detoxifying, and not as gassy as larger beans.

Once you are ready to go on a detox program, you will know what foods to eat, which will help you stay full and keep you on program.

6 HOME-MADE DETOX WATERS

Home-made detox waters are really a dream come true. I get bored easily and of course I want the best quality in my food and beverages, so when it comes to my morning detox routine, I like to mix it up. Prepare them the night before or on the spot, detox waters are great for glowing skin, a flat tummy, satisfying bowel movements and of course rising out of bed with that glad-to-be-alive feeling! So much healthier than anything pre-mixed. Of course you need good ingredients. As always, for detox, organic is always best! You don't want those pesticides causing a film.

Use filtered or spring water. I use all these but just in case, I always have some tap water evaporating on the counter for 24 hours to evaporate the chlorine. Some basic benefits of detox waters:

- Drinking water first thing in the morning is a key to **longevity**, flushes out the system after the 8 hours sleep where the body was working hard to heal and repair itself. Hot water is better than room temp. While it's not recommended to detox with cold, I can't help but drink some fruit waters on a hot day.

- Bitters and sours cause the liver to make bile, which gets sent to the gall bladder to break down fats, cholesterol and ease bowel movements.

- A sour flavor early in the morning also wakes you up, even without caffeine. Coffee and green tea are both bitters, they are both liver detox, however some coffee has so much caffeine it might actually stress the liver. Plus, if you add sugar and dairy to the coffee, it is no longer sour, is it?

- Promoting your body's daily eliminations of wastes is great for the complexion, the tummy, the colon as well as metabolism.

- Add a bitter flavor to you day can send signals to your brain that reduces cravings for sugar and other sweet drinks.

1. Salt: salt is nature's purifier. It cleanses and delivers minerals in the meantime. Natural salt contains dozens of minerals that help to balance electrolytes, hydrate the body, alkalize, maintain bone and muscle mass and lower blood pressure. Yes! I said lowers blood pressure. It's only when sodium chloride (table salt) imbalance magnesium and potassium that salt is an issue. Unfortunately most people are low in Magnesium (at least 50%) and even more people are deficient in Potassium (97% of Americans). Taking salt sole daily is a great way to cleanse impurities, alkalize and regulate the body's trace mineral stores. If you drink larger quantities, it's a wonderful internal colonic that can clean out the whole system.

- Here's the recipe from the Himalayan salt website: http://www.himalayancrystalsalt.com/sole-recipe.html

Making Sole

Step 1: If you remember your high school chemistry then you remember that water dissolves salt because the positive part of water molecules attracts the negative chloride ions and the negative part of water molecules attracts the positive sodium ions. The concept of making sole is based on the maximum concentration a substrate can dissolve into a solution. In English, this means if you keep adding salt to a glass of water you'll get to a point where the water reaches it's maximum saltiness – or concentrated with salt. At this point, if you continue adding salt then no more salt will dissolve and the crystals will sit at the bottom of the glass. This is the how you make salt sole. Maxi-concentrated or saturated salt water. Here's how to make it.

Place 1 inch of pink salt, preferably Original Himalayan Salt but could also be Real Salt in Mason Jar or a clean jar, with a good lid.

Add 2 to 3 inches of good quality artesian or spring water above the stones, completely covering the crystals with water. Let sit overnight.

Step 2: If you find that all the salt crystals have dissolved, then add another teaspoon of salt crystals to the water. The Salt Sole is ready when the water becomes fully saturated with salt and cannot hold any more, so you will actually see some crystals at the bottom.

The salt will no longer dissolve at this stage. Your finished Sole should resemble the photo at left. There should always be salt crystals in the jar. As you use up Salt Sole just add more water and more salt until the water is again

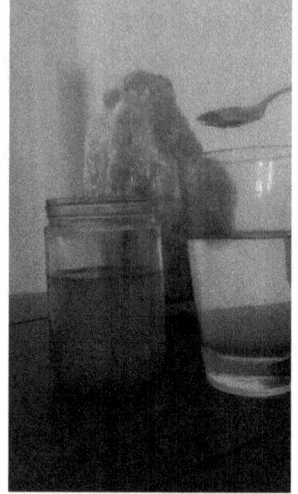

saturated. Or start over from the beginning. Remember, there should always be undissolved salt crystals on the bottom of the jar. If your salt has deeply colored flecks in there, these represent other minerals and not the sodium crystals. Therefore you still need to add more salt. The crystals are the visual proof that the water is totally concentrated with salt.

Step 3: First thing in the morning and on an empty stomach, add a teaspoon of the Salt Sole to a glass of artesian or spring water and drink. Your body will receive the frequency or vibration pattern of the Salt. Keep the jar sealed to prevent the water from evaporating either in the fridge or the cupboard. Otherwise, no special storage instructions.

A fully concentrated Salt Sole will keep forever, just like ocean water! Salt is a natural anti-bacterial and natural fungicide. It doesn't go bad or grow mold.

Drinking a teaspoon of Salt Sole in your water daily will help you with electrolyte balance, energy levels, absorption, thirst, hydration, and bowel eliminations. It is a daily practice although can also be given to constipated children or adults. Add lemon to improve the flavor – virgin margarita ☺

Diarrhea: In cases of diarrhea, triple the dose of salt sole and match that with sugar as well. Even babies can drink the homemade electrolyte beverage.

The next concept is an extension of the Salt Sole, but a strong laxative or cathartic – to be done ONLY WHEN FASTING. IT IS NOT A DAILY PRACTICE.

If you're fasting at all (meaning not eating for more than 2 days), it's necessary to do the salt flush or a laxative tea containing senna, cascara segrada, rhubarb root, etc. Check chapter 10 PRODUCTS I RECOMMEND for some of my favorite laxative teas and detox products.

Sea Salt Water Flush

Very important to use non-iodized, unbleached Sea Salt, Real Salt or Himalayan Sea Salt. Personally I love this flush. But it does involve drinking a foul salt drink, getting nauseous and then allowing a rapid evacuation of the bowels. The osmotic pressure out your back-side literally generates the feeling you are peeing out your butt. Not for everyone, but very very effective for a home-colonic.

The Salt Water Flush is an optional part of the Master Cleanse methodology, a form of fasting and detox cleansing. The longer your fast, the more important it is. The flush is used to clear out the colon, and leftover stool from the bowels particularly during the fasting stage of a detox, when solid food is not forming stool. You still need to eliminate during the detox. I only recommend you do this if you're fasting for longer than 2 days. If you're not fasting (no solid food) for longer than 2 days, the bowel movements will not be disrupted and therefore the point of the routine is reduced.

SALT FLUSH MUST BE DONE ON AN EMPTY STOMACH.

You do this by rapidly ingesting a quart of salt water, as rapidly as possible. I aim to keep it under 45 minutes. As this salt water is indigestible, it will not raise your blood pressure. However, being indigestible it will be rejected by the body. So the water solution moves quickly through the system, resulting in a liquid bowel movement much like a forceful diarrhea.

How to:

The Salt Water Flush recipe consists of 2 teaspoons (fine grind) uniodized sea salt in one quart of warm water. Drink first thing in the morning, on an empty stomach. DO NOT USE TABLE SALT, KOSHER SALT OR EPSOM SALT!!!!

Afterward, lie down on your right side for 30 minutes, helping the fluid to leave the stomach more completely and flow into the small intestine.

Because the solution is difficult to drink, here are some tips for getting it down:

- drink in a chug-a-lug fashion without pausing.

- hold your nose while swallowing so you won't smell it.

- use a straw

- Instead of using pure water add the salt to lemon water or ginger tea. Note: I am not sure this will work but have read it as a possibility.

Remain at home. When you least expect it, an urgent and recurrent movement of the bowels should occur in one – 2 hours.

Some people find it doesn't work the first and need to repeat it a second and third day. Some people have to add an extra teaspoon of salt.

If you would like to read more on Salt Flushing; there are some thoughtful pieces on the internet:

- http://www.allaboutfasting.com/salt-water-flush.html
- http://www.themastercleanse.org/salt-water-flush/

Detox waters, continued: So not all detox waters are the Salt Water Flush. Here are some other amazing detox waters to perk you up, improve regularity and flush you out. You can drink these any day of the cleanse, depending on your preferences.

Here are my top faves but you could combine most any detoxifying ingredients in water for a healthy detox!

3. **Schizandra berry soak** – The babies contain all 5 flavors. Don't expect sweet to predominate, they are spicy, salt, bitter-sweet. Put a teaspoon of dried berries into water in the evening. The next morning drink the water. Zinger!!!! And you are up and alive!

4. **Hot lemon water**— boil water as if you are making tea. Squeeze fresh lemon into the water at the end so not to destroy the vitamin C antioxidants. If you're lemon is organic then soak the slice in the water as you drink and eat the whole rind at the end. That's what I do to get extra medicine from your drink. The peel is actually high in anti-allergy citrus flavonoids, essential oils and fiber.

Turn a plain hot lemon water into a **hot spicy mama,** by tossing these things in at the end:
*a dash of cayenne pepper
*a black pepper clove
*a ginger slice
*a turmeric slice
So warming for freezing days and a great lung tonic.

5. This is a take on the traditional **Master Cleanse** which is 1 quart filtered water, 4 tablespoons darkest Grade Maple Syrup (B or C), Juice of 4 lemons, Cayenne pepper to taste. Drink hot or room temperature.

6. **Methi water**. Overnight soak 5 almonds, 1 peppercorns and 1 teaspoon of fenugreek seeds in 16 oz of water. This Ayurvedic weight loss drink great for relieving water retention, controlling blood sugar and boosting metabolism. Post-partum magic.

7. **Bitter water**. The water you've had sitting out so to remove the chlorine. Have a glass with some local or Angostura bitters– the herb gentian is the most bitter herb on the planet and a wonderful cholagogue, which means it rids the body of cholesterol. Don't save bitters for the bar. Turn them into virgin cocktails, add to seltzer and especially to dress up plain water.

8. **Apple cider water**. Unfiltered, cold-pressed. My Dad used to put it in our orange juice when we had sore throats. Cuts the mucous generated from the orange juice that's for sure. These days I add a splash of it to room

temperature water. Great for weight loss, low stomach acid, H Pylori and water retention.

9. **Dandelion and chicory root coffee substitute**. As easy as making instant coffee, this bitter bev even tastes like the real thing with its roasted flavor. Other grain coffees on the market may or may not be healthy for you, depending on the way the grains were treated and your own health status. For instance don't take Postum if you're sensitive to gluten. I have been known to drink mugs and mugs of Inka.

10. **Sangria water**. Most detox waters focus on the liver but a kidney flush is also a refreshing summer drink. This drink is so good it's worth making a pitcher. Add 1 quart of water, 3 apple slices, 2 sprigs mint, 5 juniper seeds and 3 cucumber slices. That's some gourmet water. Kids will love it too!

Just because you put fruit into water, doesn't mean it's detoxifying so let me know what other combos you've come up with. I'll test them out.

7 RECIPES FOR DETOX

Shakes and Smoothies

1. Liquid Lunch:

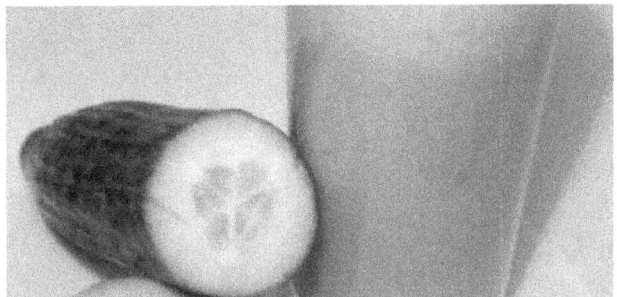

¼ cup organic carrot juice (substitute with other vegetable juice)

½ avocado

1 cup sunflower sprouts

½ organic apple, cored (or ½ cucumber)

½ lemon, squeezed

1 tsp spirulina or chlorella (optional)

1 clove garlic (optional)

Directions
Note: If you have a juicer, juice the carrots first, as fresh juice is always better.

Pour the juice into the blender. Add rest of the ingredients into the blender. Blend until smooth. Pour over ice or drink at room temperature. This juice is energizing, refreshing, detoxifying and satisfying. Most importantly it's packed with vitamins, minerals, some proteins and healthy fats. It's a meal of its own or on the side of a detoxifying quinoa or brown rice salad, hot or cold.

2. Green Magi

2 cups fresh spinach
2 cups almond milk, unsweetened

1 large apple, cored, any variety

1 kiwi fruit

⅓ chia seeds

1 tablespoon coconut oil

1/2 teaspoon ground cinnamon

DIRECTIONS

1. Soak chia seeds in almond milk for 10 minutes.

2. Blend spinach and almond milk until smooth.

3. Add remaining ingredients, and blend until smooth. Enjoy!

Use frozen fruit to make smoothie cold.

    3.   Cleanser Shake

In the Juicer Press: You could Blend these with a Vitamix, core the apple in this case.

1 Green apple

½ Lemon

2 large carrots

1 beet

1 inch ginger

Optional Directions:

**Blend or Stir in 1 tablespoon olive oil and 1 tablespoon of flax seed powder into the fresh pressed juice.

Porridge alternative to brown rice

Chia Seed Pudding

Ingredients

1.5 cups Coconut water (optional, use apple sauce)

1 Tbsp raw honey or maple syrup

1 tsp carob powder (optional)

1/4 tsp cinnamon

1/4 cup chia seeds

Coconut milk (optional)

Directions:

- Combine coconut water, honey, vanilla and cinnamon in a sealable container (like a mason jar!)
- Seal and shake vigorously
- Add chia seeds and shake again
- Wait about 30 minutes for them to set up.
- Can warm up or eat at room temperature
- Add coconut milk on top if desired

Broth

Potassium Broth: While bone broths are healthy and nourishing, vegetarian broths are key to reduce blood pressure, balance electrolytes and hydration. In a pot of filtered boiling water add a handful of organic carrots, 3 yukon gold potatoes, 1 white or yellow onion and a tsp of Salt sole or ¼ tsp of Himalayan, Real or unbleached sea salt. Simmer until veggies are cooked. Drink alone or veggies. Take it after exercise instead of coconut water and on fasting days.

Bone Broth:
Ingredients

- 3-4 pounds beef marrow and knuckle bone

- 2 pounds meaty bones such as short ribs
- ½ cup raw apple cider vinegar
- 1 whole lemon, with peel, cut
- 4 quarts filtered water
- 3 celery stalks, halved
- 3 carrots, halved
- 3 onions, quartered
- Handful of fresh parsley
- Sea salt

Method
1. Place bones in a pot or a crockpot, add apple cider vinegar, lemon and water, and let the mixture sit for 1 hour so the acids can leach the mineral out of the bones.
2. Add more water if needed to cover the bones.
3. Add the vegetables bring to a boil and skim the scum from the top and discard.
4. Reduce to a low simmer, cover, and cook for 24-72 hours (if you're not comfortable leaving the pot to simmer overnight, turn off the heat and let it sit overnight, then turn it back on and let simmer all day the next day)
5. During the last 10 minutes of cooking, throw in a handful of fresh parsley for added flavor and minerals.
6. Let the broth cool and strain it, making sure all marrow is knocked out
7. of the marrow bones and into the broth.
8. Add sea salt to taste and drink the broth as is or store in fridge up to 5 to 7 days or freezer up to 6 months for use in soups or stews

Dips

1. Tahini

Here is a recipe to make Tahini using only Sesame seeds and olive oil:

- 16 oz sesame seeds (lightly toast on dry stovetop if desired)
- 3/ 4 cup virgin olive oil
- Options for other ingredients. You could also blend fresh parsley or Tarragon or arugula into it.

Directions:

1. Add all ingredients into blender and blend until smooth. Tahini tastes great in dips, dressings, smoothies and sauces.

2. You can use it to make a dipping sauce, adding fresh lemon juice, Angostura bitters, cayenne.

3. Sprouted Hummus:

Soak 2 cups of dried chickpeas in a bowl of water over night, drain and rinse before using. If you have an extra day, put the chick peas in a mason jar or clear bowl. Rinse every 4-6 hours to keep peas moist. When a tail sprouts, they are ready to use and eat. Also a delicious snack!

Substitution Tips: Add fresh herbs, spices and use different nut butters (sunflower seed butter, pumpkin seed butter or almond butter) to change the flavor

INGREDIENTS: In a food processor, blend:

- 2 cups of soaked chickpeas
- 2 cloves raw garlic, chopped
- 3 tablespoons of tahini (sesame butter)
- Juice from 1 lemon (approx. 3-4 tablespoons)
- ½ teaspoon roasted cumin seeds or powder
- Olive oil (for moisture, as desired)

- 2 tablespoons chopped, fresh parsley (optional)

For best flavor, let sit over night

Eat with raw veggies; zucchini, carrots, celery, broccoli, mushrooms, cauliflower, etc.

4. Almond Sauce

- 2 tablespoons of organic almond butter
- Juice from a lime
- 1 clove garlic, crushed or finely chopped
- 1 teaspoon miso
- 1 tablespoon of boiled water
- 1 teaspoon olive oil
- Optional 1 teaspoon chopped parsley or cilantro

Directions

Whisk miso into hot water

Stir into bowl with almond butter

Mix remaining ingredients

5. Arugula Pistou (pesto without the cheese)

- 4 cups of packed fresh arugula (preferably organic, not moldy)
- 1 tablespoon freshly minced garlic (2-3 cloves)- let sit for 10 minutes
- 2 tablespoons chopped raw walnuts plus 1 tablespoon
- 1 cup of extra virgin olive oil
- Dash of pepper and cayenne each to taste
- 1/8 teaspoon powdered vitamin C (optional) or juice from ½ small lemon

Prepare an ice water bath in a large bowl and bring a large pot of water to a boil. Put the arugula in a fine mesh strainer or sieve and plunge it into the boiling water. Immediately immerse the arugula and stir so that it blanches evenly. Remove after 15 second. Shake off excess water and then plunge the arugula into the ice bath and stir again so it cools as fast as possible. Drain well.

Squeeze the water out of the arugula with your hands until very dry. Roughly chop the arugula and put it into the blender/Vitamix. Add the garlic, pepper and cayenne to taste, olive oil, 2 tablespoon walnuts and the vitamin C, if using. Blend for at least 30 seconds.

If have not used vitamin C, squeeze juice from half a lemon into the mixture at the end. Will keep several days in a tightly sealed container. Before serving add remaining walnuts on top.

Salads – eat with brown rice

1. Grapefruit and Avocado Salad

Ingredients

- Grate fresh beet or use boiled beets
- 1 whole grapefruit, peeled – it's better if inside skins are peeled
- 1 ripe avocado
- Finely chopped onion to taste
- 2 tablespoons olive oil
- Juice from ½ grapefruit or lemon

Directions: slice avocado thinly and delicately peel the grapefruit sections. Toss ingredients with Olive oil and Grapefruit juice.

2. Watercress and Beet Salad

- 4 medium-sized beets
- 1/2 cup apple cider vinegar
- 1 tablespoon grape seed oil
- 4 small carrots, peeled and cut on the diagonal, 1/4-inch thick
- 2 tablespoons raw pumpkin seeds
- 1 bunch watercress, washed and well-dried, bunch separated and thick stems removed
- 3 radishes, thinly sliced
- Freshly ground pepper

- Extra-virgin olive oil

Directions

Place beets in a medium-sized saucepan with the vinegar. Fill with water to cover. Cover with tin foil. Poke 4 holes in foil. Cook until beets are tender (a knife can easily pierce through), about 45 minutes. Allow beets to cool, then cut each into 8 wedges. Chill in refrigerator.
Pour a tablespoon of oil into a hot saute pan. Add the carrots and cook until golden brown on one side (medium-high heat). Add sugar and stir, cooking until tender and crispy, about 5-7 minutes. Allow carrots to cool a bit, then chill in refrigerator.
Put the watercress in a salad bowl. Add the radishes, beets, and carrots. Season with fresh herbs, freshly ground pepper, and a drizzle of olive oil.
Toast pumpkin seeds in toaster oven or on stove top until golden. Top the salad

3. Seed Salad

Ingredients:

- 1 whole pomegranate, deseeded
- 1 tablespoon extra-virgin olive oil
- 1 Sprig fresh mint leaves, pulled
- 1/8 tsp mustard seeds
- 1/8 cumin seeds

Directions:

Lightly toast seeds in a dry pan

Mix all items together in a bowl.

Kitchari (cleansing staple)

for your constitution (Kapha/Pitta)

Ingredients

- 1/2 cup brown rice

  1 cup Lentils or split peas

  6 cups (approx.) Water

  1/2 to 1 inch Ginger Root, chopped or grated

  a bit of Mineral Salt (1/4 tsp. or so)

  2 tsp. Coconut oil or Red Palm Oil

  1/2 tsp. Coriander Powder

  1/2 tsp. Cumin Powder

  1/2 tsp. Whole Cumin Seeds

  ½ tsp Mustard Seeds

  1/2 tsp. Turmeric Powder

  1 pinch Asafoetida (Hing)

  Handful Fresh Cilantro Leaves

  1 and 1/2 cups Assorted Fresh Vegetables (Whatever you've purchased)

Kitchari means mixture, usually of two grains. This is one kitchari recipe that is particularly nourishing and easy to digest. Please note the options below for some alternatives.

Options. If you know your Ayurvedic constitution you can tailor it for you. Vata is earth. Pitta is fire. Kapha is water.

Vegetables such as zucchini,
asparagus, sweet potato
For Vata or Kapha conditions:
add a pinch of ginger powder

For Pitta: leave out the mustard seeds

Preparation

Carefully pick over rice and lentils to remove any stones. Wash each separately in at least 2 changes of water. Add the 6 cups of water to the rice and lentils and cook covered until it becomes soft, about 20 minutes.

While that is cooking, prepare any vegetables that suit your constitution. Cut them into smallish pieces. Add the vegetables to the cooked rice and dal mixture and cook 10 minutes longer.

In a separate saucepan, sauté the seeds in the coconut or red palm oil until they pop. Then add the other spices. Stir together to release the flavors. Stir the sautéed spices into the cooked lentils, rice, and vegetable mixture. Add the mineral salt and chopped fresh cilantro and serve.

Caution: Kitchari mono-diet can lead to constipation if taken exclusively for several days, as it is low in fiber. To ensure proper elimination, the following may prove helpful if taken once a day, away from kitchari meals: psyllium husks or flax or chia seeds with water OR oat bran OR prune juice.

8 SUPPLEMENTS

These supplements are all beneficial for detoxifying, methylation, resetting genes, clearing out waste products such as old hormones and pesticide metabolites, heavy metals, old stool and drug metabolites. To increase the effect of any detox, I recommend seeking qualified advice over which supplements are right for you. This is not an exhaustive list , but it is a list of important organ detoxifying agents. Remember, not all brands are equal, so get a recommendation or look at the website I recommend at www.milliesays.com.

I have been recommending a 7 DAY NUTRACLEAN CLEANSING SYSTEM available here: HTTP://WWW.NUTRAMETRIX.COM/EATINGFORMEANING but many other supplements can be used for detox. Use my email MILLIELYTLE@GMAIL.COM apply code 10OFFMA at checkout for a 10% discount on Nutrametrix and Market America products. I do make commissions on these products, and it helps me continue my business so I thank you for your trust.

AMINO ACIDS:

- DMG, NAC, MSM, SAMe

ACTIVATED B COMPLEX ESPECIALLY

- B3, B6, B12, Folic Acid

PHYTONUTIRENTS:

- Indol-3-Carbinol (I-3-C) with DIM from broccoli and cabbage for hormone detox

- OPC-3 from grape seed, maritime pine bark, bilberry and resveratrol

HERBS

- Liver Detox: Dandelion, Burdock, Turmeric, Yellow Dock

- Kidney: Parsley, Juniper, Cranberry

- Colon: Rhubarb, Cascara Segrada, Psyllium, Aloe

Food Based Fruit and Vegetable Supplements:

- Juice + anti-inflammatory, detox and food

MINERALS:

- Magnesium, Zinc, Calcium-D-Glucarate

PECTINS:

- Apple Pectin, Modified Citrus Pectin

Seaweeds:

- Spirulina, Chlorella, E3 Live, Kelp

SULPHUR CONTAINING (Not the same as Sulfa):

- DIM, I-3-C, Aged Garlic, Sulforaphane

Probiotics

- Support immunity, gut health and integrity, gut-brain connection and mood, digestion and elimination of bacteria, fungus and other microbiome disturbing the gut flora.

- Found in sauerkraut, organic yogurt, kombucha and other fermented foods. Also available in TABLET, capsule, powder and with DIGESTIVE ENZYMES.

- Colostrum, liquid gold from a cow's udder. Not so much for detox but afterwards to rebuilding a leaky gut. You might be able to eat foods you couldn't before after a year on Colostrum and effective Probiotics.

9 COMING OFF THE DETOX

If you are working on your relationship to food, it is important to add foods back into your diet gradually. This stage can get complicated and confusing. I recommend working with me or another qualified Naturopathic Doctor or Nutritionist to guide you. The first reason is that you don't want to shock your system into feeling upset again. The second reason is that this is a perfect opportunity to reintroduce other foods into your diet and observe how they react in your system. Depending on your nutritional and health goals, the process of reintroduction can take a while, weeks, in fact. While the reintroduction schedule below outlines 22 days, if you have many reactions, this can be delayed substantially.

The key point to remember is to re- introduce only one food at a time, every 3 days. After you have found that a substance is agreeable with you, it may be combined with other foods you are tolerating well. If the substance disagrees you must wait until all reactions are reduced before introducing a new food. Also the realization that one food or food group is producing a sensitivity reaction means there may be other questions asked that takes time to be resolved. E.g. If you are sensitive to oats, is it gluten-free oats as well or only oats contaminated with gluten. This could take and extra 6 days to determine.

CONTINUE TO DO THE FOLLOWING:
- No canned products.
- Eat raw fruit. Eat fruit by itself: 1/2 before or 2 hours after eating.
- Drink liquids 1/2 hour before or 1 hour after eating for better digestion

YOU MAY CHOOSE TO ADD ANY OF THESE INGREDIENTS IN THE FOLLOWING TIME FRAMES. ONCE YOU FIND THAT YOU TOLERATE

THEM WELL YOU MAY CONTINUE TO USE THEM.

Coming off the Detox Diet

It is important to add foods back into your diet gradually. The first reason is that you don't want to shock your system into feeling upset again. The second reason is that this is a perfect opportunity to reintroduce other foods into your diet and observe how they react in your system.

The key point to remember is to introduce only one substance at a time, within a 3 day period as some reactions can be delayed. After you have found that a substance is agreeable with you, it may be combined with other foods you are tolerating well

CONTINUE TO DO THE FOLLOWING:
No canned products.
Eat raw fruit. Eat fruit by itself: 1/2 before or 2 hours after eating
Drink liquids 1/2 hour before or 1 hour after eating for better digestion

YOU MAY CHOOSE TO ADD ANY OF THESE INGREDIENTS IN THE FOLLOWING TIME FRAMES. ONCE YOU FIND THAT YOU TOLERATE THEM WELL YOU MAY CONTINUE TO USE THEM.

*********When you introduce a food. Eat 3 servings of it in one day, in forms that you normally would include in your diet.

DAY 1-4

100% yeast free rye bread
Amaranth
avocadoes (great with sandwiches)
bananas
Buckwheat/Kasha
Dairy-free ice-cream (e.g. rice dream)
honey (raw unpasteurized)
Millet
mushrooms
Organic Canola oil
Organic Corn, corn oil

organic dried fruit
Quinoa and quinoa pasta
Rice pasta/rice noodles
Safflower oil
Sesame oil
organic Strawberries
Sunflower oil
tomato sauce (without sugar and preservatives)
Wheat free soya sauce
Wheat-free/gluten free bread

(No hydrogenated, fractionated oils, margarine or butter spread)

DAY 5-7

Almond butter	Brazil nuts	Tahini spread
Almond milk	Hazelnuts	Walnuts
(unsweetened)	Pecans	
Almonds	Sesame seeds	

(no peanuts, peanut butter, macadamia nus or pistachios)

DAY 8-10

	Salmon	necessary to have
Cod	Sardines	tuna and salmon
Halibut	Trout	from cans use
Herring	White fish (no	Albacore tuna
Mackerel	shellfish), if it is	canned in water

DAY 11-14

Chicken	Eggs	Turkey
Duck	Lamb	

(organic meets and free-range eggs are preferred)

DAY 15-18

Lentils
Beans:

adzuki	fava	pinto
barley	kidney	red
black	lima	Split peas
black-eyed peas	mung	white
Chickpeas	navy	

(make sure to soak and rinse your beans, peas before cooking)

Grains:
kamut	Spelt

DAY 19-20

Feta Cheese   Gee   Yogurt

DAY 21

Whole grain products (bread, pasta, baked goods)

DAY 22

rennet-free whole raw-milk cow cheese (unpasteurized)

10 PRODUCTS I RECOMMEND

Here are links to products I have discussed, recommend and use myself. Disclosure: I do make affiliate fees from Amazon.com See my website at www.eatingformeaning.com for more health products.

100% Yeast Free Rye or Pumperknickel Bread:
http://www.amazon.com/Mestemacher-Pumpernickel-17-6-Ounce-Packages-Pack/dp/B000LKVFBM

Bob's Red Mill Gluten-Free Products:
http://www.amazon.com/Bobs-Red-Mill-Gluten-Free-All-Purpose/dp/B000KEPBCS

Nutrametrix Professional Supplements:
http://www.nutrametrix.com/eatingformeaning/?refEmail=203F2F072C
3C212F370720392A3B220229572E392E

Dry Skin Brush: http://www.amazon.com/gp/product/B000KNHJ5G

Himalayan Salt Inhaler:
http://www.amazon.com/gp/product/B00C2GZPJ6 or
http://www.amazon.com/gp/product/B006U41QN0

Himalayan Salt: http://www.himalayancrystalsalt.com/sole-recipe.html

Juice +: Whole foods supplement
http://lgould.juiceplus.com/content/JuicePlus/en.html#.VV3fe_lViko

Laxative Teas:
Yogi Soothing Mint 6 pack:
http://www.amazon.com/gp/product/B000CMF17S OR
Traditional Medicinals Organic Move Out
http://www.amazon.com/gp/product/B0009F3PJE OR
Triple Leaf Herbal Laxative
http://www.amazon.com/gp/product/B0007DHMK6

ABOUT THE AUTHOR

Millennia Ruth Lytle, affectionately known as Dr. Millie, is a licensed Naturopathic Doctor and Certified Nutrition Specialist with a special interest in solving health puzzles, naturally. She "fills gaps of care your doctor doesn't" with Naturopathic Medicine and custom-made nutrition programs. She is a member of **Tournesol Wellness** Primary Care Team and works in tandem with the medical team to improve primary care in New York. She is a "doctorpreneur" incorporating science-based Nutrametrix supplementation into her programs. She has a goal of living until 120 years old and invites you on her journey.

She is the founder the Food for Mood Diet and the year-long nutrition program, Eating for Meaning (EfM) that helps YOU heal your relationship to food; prevent and treat chronic health problems using all-natural methods. She has a passion for helping you return your body to normal function.

She has a goal of living until a healthy age of 120 years old and invites you to join her because anti-aging is more than vanity, it is the prevention and treatment of chronic illness.

She lives and practices in New York. You can reach her at www.eatingformeaning.com

www.ingramcontent.com/pod-product-compliance
Lightning Source LLC
Chambersburg PA
CBHW071000290526
45795CB00005B/1719